Copyright 2023

All right reserved.No part of this book should be reproduced without express permission of the author.

Reproduction of all or any part of this book is punishable unders relevant law.

Table of Contents

Bronchitis is an inflammation of the lining of your bronchial tubes, which carry air to and from your lungs. People who have bronchitis often cough up thickened mucus, which can be discolored. Bronchitis may be either acute or chronic.

Often developing from a cold or other respiratory infection, acute bronchitis is very common. Chronic bronchitis, a more serious condition, is a constant irritation or inflammation of the lining of the bronchial tubes, often due to smoking.

Acute bronchitis, also called a chest cold, usually improves within a week to 10 days without lasting effects, although the cough may linger for weeks.

However, if you have repeated bouts of bronchitis, you may have chronic bronchitis, which requires medical attention. Chronic bronchitis is one of the conditions included in chronic

obstructive pulmonary disease (COPD).

BREAKFAST

1. Blueberry Banana Baked Oatmeal

Prep Time: 15 Minutes

Cook Time: 40 Minutes

Servings: 2

Ingredients

- 2 tbsp ground chia or ground flax
- 6 tbsp water
- 2 cup gluten-free oats
- 2 tbsp coconut sugar or brown sugar
- 2 tsp cinnamon
- 1/4 tsp nutmeg
- 1/4 tsp cardamom
- 1 tsp baking powder
- 3/4 tsp sea salt
- 3/4 cup pecans
- 1 3/4 cup almond milk
- 1/3 cup maple syrup

- 1/4 cup coconut oil melted
- 2 tsp vanilla extract
- 1 cup banana mashed
- 2 cups blueberries fresh or frozen

Instructions

1. Preheat oven to 350F/176C. Make chia egg by combining ground chia with water. Stir well to combine and let sit at least 5 mins.
2. In a large mixing bowl combine oats, coconut sugar, cinnamon, nutmeg, cardamom, baking powder and sea salt. Reserve 2 tbsp pecans for topping and add the rest. Mix to combine.
3. In a separate smaller mixing bowl, combine wet ingredients: chia egg, almond milk, maple syrup, melted coconut oil, vanilla extract. Mix to combine.
4. Add mashed banana to dry bowl, then pour in wet ingredients and stir to combine.
5. Reserve 1/2 cup blueberries for topping, and add the remaining to the bottom of your baking dish (I used a square 8.5x8.5 inch baking dish). Slowly pour oatmeal mixture overtop and spread to even. Top oatmeal bake with 1/2 cup reserved blueberries, and 2 tbsp

reserved pecans. (Optional to also top with sliced banana if you have, but not necessary).

6. Bake oatmeal for 40-50 minutes or until golden and firm. Let cool for at least 15 minutes to set. Then cut in squares and serve. (I like to serve with coconut yogurt, fresh banana and maple syrup).

Prep Time: 30 Minutes

Cook Time: 15 Minutes

Servings: 16

Ingredients

Wet Ingredients:

- 1 cup vegan butter melted
- 3/4 cup pumpkin puree canned
- 3/4 cup brown sugar
- 1/4 cup cane sugar
- 1/4 cup maple syrup
- 1 tsp vanilla extract

Dry Ingredients:

- 2 cups all purpose flour
- 1 1/3 cup old fashioned rolled oats
- 1 tbsp flaxseed meal or chia meal
- 1 tbsp pumpkin spice
- 1 tsp cinnamon
- 1 tsp baking soda
- 1/4 tsp sea salt

- 3/4 cup semi-sweet chocolate chips

Instructions

1. In a large mixing bowl add the wet ingredients; melted vegan butter, pumpkin puree, brown sugar, cane sugar, maple syrup, vanilla extract. Mix well to combine.

2. In a separate smaller bowl combine the flour, oats, flaxseed meal, pumpkin spice, cinnamon, baking soda, and sea salt. Mix together.

3. Add the dry ingredients to the wet in batches, folding into the cookie dough batter until just combined. Then fold in the chocolate chips. Cover with a tea towel and refrigerate for 20 to 30 minutes, or until the dough has chilled and thickened into scoopable cookie dough.

4. Preheat the oven to 350F/180C and line three baking trays with parchment paper. Scoop 2 tablespoons of cookie dough batter onto the tray to form a cookie shape, until you've used all the dough (about 6 large cookies per tray). Bake for 15 minutes, let cool for 5 minutes, then transfer to a cooling rack to cool completely.

NOTES

1. Letting the dough sit for 20 to 30 minutes gives optimal time for the oats to absorb the liquid for an easier-to-scoop cookie dough batter.

2. This cookie dough is more wet than traditional cookie dough, and that's okay. You won't be able to roll it in a ball like traditional dough, but use a tablespoon to scoop and form a cookie shape on your baking tray.

3. Let your cookies cool entirely before eating for a non-cakey texture. The longer they sit, the less cakey they become.

4. Like most oatmeal cookies, these cookies get even better over time! These cookies will keep for up to 5 days. Transfer to an air-tight container and keep at room temperate for 3 days or stored in the fridge for 5 days.

Prep Time: 10 Minutes

Cook Time: 25 Minutes

Servings: 12

Ingredients

- 1 1/2 cups unsweetened almond milk
- 1/4 cup mashed banana (1/2 medium banana)
- 1/4 cup coconut flour
- 1 cup gluten-free baking flour
- 2 tbsp natural peanut butter
- 1 tbsp maple syrup (more for serving)
- 1 tsp baking powder
- 1/4 tsp baking soda
- pinch sea salt
- splash coconut oil or olive oil, for greasing
- strawberry chia jam optional for serving

Instructions

1. In a high-speed blender, combine the almond milk, mashed banana, coconut flour, gluten-free baking

flour, natural peanut butter, maple syrup, baking powder, baking soda and sea salt. Blend until smooth.

2. Lightly grease a large non-stick skillet with coconut oil over medium heat. Give the batter a good stir, then pour the batter into the pan in 2 heaping tablespoon portions, cooking 2 or 3 at a time. Cook until little tiny bubbles cover the surface of the pancakes and the bottom is golden brown, about 2 minutes. Flip and continue to cook until also golden brown on the bottom, about 2 minutes more. Add more oil to the pan as needed to keep the pancakes from sticking.

3. To keep pancakes warm while cooking: Preheat oven to 200F/100C. Transfer the pancakes to the prepared baking sheet and keep warm in the oven while you cook the remaining pancakes.

Prep Time: 20 Minutes

Cook Time: 40 Minutes

Servings: 12

Ingredients

- 1 baguette (400g or about 10 cups) preferably one day-old
- Custard:
- 1 can coconut milk (400 ml/13.5 fl. oz)
- 14 oz silken tofu (1 block)
- ½ cup coconut sugar or brown sugar
- 2 tbsp vegan butter
- 2 tbsp corn starch
- 2 tsp pure vanilla extract

Crumble Topping:

- 1 tsp cinnamon
- ¼ cup all purpose flour
- 1/3 sup coconut sugar or brown sugar
- 2 tbsp vegan butter
- ¼ cup pecans chopped

- 1 apple thinly sliced (optional)

Instructions

1. Cut day-old baguette into bite sized squares. (Alternatively, you can use fresh baguette, spread out the pieces onto a baking tray and let "dry out" for at least 2 hours).

2. In a blender, combine the coconut milk, tofu, coconut sugar, butter, corn starch, vanilla and cinnamon. Blend until smooth.

3. Transfer bread bites to a large rectangular baking dish (8 x 11 inches) pour in the creamy custard and press down with your hands gently to soak everything. Cover and refrigerate overnight.

4. Preheat oven to 350F/176C. In a small bowl combine the flour, sugar and vegan butter. Massage with your finger tips to create a crumble texture. Sprinkle in the pecans and mix again.

5. Sprinkle the crumble topping over the French toast casserole and tuck sliced apples into the nook sand crannies if using. Bake for 40 minutes, or until golden on top. Let cool slightly, cut into squares and serve with maple syrup.

6. French toast casserole will keep for up to 5 days. Store in the fridge in an air-tight container.

Prep Time: 20 Minutes

Cook Time: 40 Minutes

Servings: 8

Ingredients

- 2 lbs rhubarb , fresh or frozen, chopped
- 1 lb strawberries , chopped
- 1 cup raw cane sugar
- 3 tbsp corn starch , or arrowroot powder
- 1 tbsp lime , or lemon
- 1 tsp vanilla extract

Oat Topping:

- 1 cup gluten-free oats
- 1/2 cup almond flour (ground blanched almonds)
- 1/2 cup sliced almonds
- 1/4 cup raw cane sugar , or coconut sugar
- 1/2 tsp cinnamon
- 1/4 tsp cardamon , optional
- pinch sea salt
- 1/3 cup coconut oil , melted

Instructions

1. Preheat oven to 350F/175C. In a large mixing bowl combine the rhubarb, strawberries, sugar, corn starch, lime and vanilla extract. Mix together to combine. Let sit for 10 minutes.

2. In a separate smaller mixing bowl combine the oats, almond flour, shaved almonds, sugar, cinnamon, cardamom, and sea salt. Stir to combine. Pour in the melted coconut oil and mix together.

3. In a 9x6 baking dish, pour in the sweet fruity mixture. Sprinkle with the crumble topping in an even layer. Bake for 45 minutes to 1 hour. Or, until the fruity sides are thick and bubbly, and the top is golden brown. Let rest for 20 minutes before serving. Serve warm or at room temperature, optional to serve with vegan ice cream or coconut yogurt.

4. Crisp will keep in fridge for up to one week.

Prep Time: 30 Minutes

Cook Time: 20 Minutes

Servings: 8

Ingredients

Dry Ingredients:

- 2 cups all-purpose flour or gluten-free flour blend, plus more for sprinkling
- 1 cup gluten-free oats , plus more for sprinkling
- 1/3 cup cane sugar , plus more for sprinkling
- 1 tbsp ground chia or ground flax
- 2 tbsp baking powder
- 1/2 tsp baking soda
- 1/2 tsp sea salt finely ground
- 1/4 tsp ground cardamom optional

Wet Ingredients

- 3/4 cup Liberte coconut yogurt plain
- 1/2 cup almond milk
- 1 tsp vanilla extract
- The Rest:

- 1/2 cup vegan butter chilled

- 1 cup frozen wild blueberries or fresh

- 2 tbsp almond milk

- 1 tbsp neutral oil

Glaze (Optional)

- 1/4 cup Liberte coconut yogurt

- 2 tsp lemon juice

- 1 1/2 tsp agave

Instructions

1. Preheat oven to 375F/190C. Sift all-purpose flour through a fine mesh sieve into a large mixing bowl. (Optional to sift twice for extra light scones). Pulse oats in a blender, until finely ground, and add to bowl along with cane sugar, ground chia, baking powder, baking soda, sea salt and cardamom. Mix lightly to combine.

2. In a separate bowl combine coconut yogurt, almond milk and vanilla extract. Mix well.

3. Cut cold vegan butter into small cubes and add to dry ingredients. Massage with fingertips to combine the dough and butter, turning into a shaggy dough. Don't

overwork the dough here, it should be shaggy and loosely combined. It's okay if it looks a little dry.

4. Slowly pour in liquid ingredients, while gently stirring to combine. Again, don't over mix. It's okay to be dry in places. Next add blueberries and mix gently to just combine.

5. Turn dough onto clean work surface and form together to make a round disk, about 1-inch thick. Optional to sprinkle the top with more flour if there are sticky spots while forming.

6. In a small bowl, whisk together almond milk and neutral oil. Paint the surface with liquid mixture to cover, and sprinkle with oats and cane sugar.

7. Line a baking tray with parchment paper. Using a spatula gently transfer scones to baking tray. Leave space between to allow them to grow. Bake for 20-25 minutes, or until golden.

8. For the glaze (optional): combine yogurt, lemon juice and agave. Drizzle scones with glaze and serve.

9. Scones will keep for 3 days, but best served fresh.

Prep Time: 20 Minutes

Cook Time: 40 Minutes

Servings: 5

Ingredients

- 2 zucchinis (230g each)
- 1 small sweet potato (200g)
- olive oil to spray
- For The "Egg Whites" Sauce:
- 1/2 cup raw cashews soaked overnight
- 2 tbsp nutritional yeast
- 3 cloves garlic
- 1 lemon juiced (approx. 2 tbsp)
- 1/2 cup water plus more if needed
- 1/2 tsp onion powder optional
- pinch salt

Instructions

1. Turn oven to 400F/200C. Using a fork, poke small holes in sweet potato going all the way round, about 1-

inch apart. Line baking tray with parchment paper and place sweet potato on top. Bake for 30 minutes, or until cooked through. Place to the side.

2. Spiralize zucchinis into noodles and spread onto sheets of paper towel. Place more paper towel on top and gently press the water out of zucchini as best you can.

3. In a blender add "egg whites" ingredients: soaked cashews (strained), nutritional yeast, garlic, lemon juice, water, onion powder (optional) and salt. Blend until creamy and smooth.

4. Line a baking tray with tin foil and lightly spray with olive oil. Build "egg nests" onto tray by bunching the noodles tightly together to look like a nest. (Should make about 5 nests). Pour 3 tbsp "egg whites" sauce into the centre of each egg nest. Bake nests in the oven for 10-12 minutes, or until zucchini is lightly browned.

5. Slice open sweet potato. Using a melon baller scoop the insides to form a ball. This will be your "egg yolk." Place a ball of sweet potato into the centre of each cooked nest.

6. Serve zucchini egg nests with more "egg white" sauce to drizzle.

7. Cashews must be soaked in advanced, otherwise pour boiling water over cashews in a bowl and let sit for 1 hour. If you do not have time for this you can also substitute the cashews for hemp hearts. Hemp hearts require no soaking before use.

8. Zucchinis are naturally full of water, so it's important to press out as much water as you can before baking. I do this by spreading the zucchini noodles out onto thick paper towel, place more paper towel on top and gently press the water out of zucchini as best you can.

9. Soaking the cashews and spiralizing the sweet potato noodles ahead of time will make the cook time for this recipe faster.

10. "Egg white" sauce will keep in fridge for up to one week. Use as a dressing for buddha bowls, or as alfredo sauce in my Sweet Potato Alfredo.

Prep Time: 35 Minutes

Cook Time: 15 Minutes

Servings: 5

Ingredients

Crust:

- 1 cup gluten-free rolled oats
- 1/4 cup shredded coconut
- 3/4 cup almond flour (ground blanched almonds)
- 1/2 tsp cinnamon
- 1/4 tsp salt
- 1/4 cup coconut oil
- 3 tbsp agave

Filling:

- 3/4 cup raw cashews soaked overnight, strained
- 1/4 can coconut milk
- 8 tsp agave
- 2 tbsp coconut yogurt
- 1 lemon juiced
- 1/2 tsp vanilla extract

- pinch salt

Instructions

1. In a food processor add oats, pulse until it's a flour-like substance. Then add shredded coconut, almond flour, cinnamon and salt. Melt coconut oil in saucepan on medium-high heat, add agave and stir to combine. Pour liquid mixture into food processor and blend until combined, and mixture is a dough-like substance.
2. Create tart shells by pressing the dough mixture into the bottom of the tart pans and up the sides, to be about 1/2 cm thick. (I used five, 4-inch tart pans with removable bottoms, but you can modify depending on what you have. See notes below on tart pans).
3. Preheat oven to 350F/175C and bake crust for 8-10 minutes, or until golden in colour. Let cool.
4. In a blender add soaked cashews (strained), coconut milk, agave, coconut yogurt, lemon juice, vanilla extract, and salt. Blend to combine.
5. Pour filling into the centre of each tart. Then, gently tap against work surface to release any air bubbles. Place in freezer for approx. 1 hour, or until solid.

6. When ready to eat, remove tarts from freezer and let thaw 15 minutes before slicing. Optional to top with your favourite fruits (I used blueberries and sliced kiwi).

Prep Time: 10 Minutes

Cook Time: 15 Minutes

Servings: 4

Ingredients

- 2 tsp miso white shiro
- 4 cups vegetable broth
- 1/2 tsp fresh ginger , grated
- pinch chili flakes
- 2 kaffir lime leaves
- 1 tbsp tamari
- 100 g extra firm tofu
- 1 sweet potato small (optional)
- 135 g soba noodles
- 1 bok choy (or two baby bok choy)
- 100 ml canned coconut milk
- 1/2 lime , juiced
- 2 green onion , diced (for topping)
- peanuts , chopped(for topping)
- fresh cilantro , chopped (for topping)

Instructions

1. In a small bowl add miso with a splash hot water. Whisk to combine. Then pour miso liquid into a large pot with vegetable broth, ginger, chilli flakes, lime leaves and soy sauce. Simmer for 5 minutes.

2. Chop tofu into small bite sized cubes, and spiralize sweet potato into noodles. Add tofu and sweet potato noodles to pot and simmer for 1-2 minutes. Then add soba noodles and cook for 5 minutes, or as directed on package. Chop bok choy and add to soup. Finally, pour in coconut milk and lime juice, stir to combine.

3. Divide pho into bowls and top with chopped peanuts, green onion and cilantro.

4. Whisking miso with a little bit of hot water before starting will stop it from clumping.

5. Optional to use water over vegetable broth.

Prep Time: 5 Minutes

Cook Time: 15 Minutes

Servings: 1

Ingredients

- 2 tsp coconut oil
- 1/2 zucchini chopped
- 1/2 cup purple cabbage shredded
- pinch sea salt
- 3/4 cups quinoa cooked
- 1/4 cup chickpeas cooked
- 1/2 tsp ground cumin
- 1 tsp curry powder
- 1/4 cup coconut milk
- 1/2 lemon juiced
- pinch cayenne pepper flakes (optional)
- 1/2 cup kale , chopped (or spinach)

Instructions

1. In a deep skillet add coconut oil and zucchini. Bring to medium-high heat and cook zucchini for 2-3 minutes to soften, then add cabbage and pinch salt. Cook veg for another 5-6 minutes until cabbage has slightly softened.

2. Add quinoa and chickpeas to the skillet and toss. Season with cumin and curry powder, and pour in coconut milk and lemon juice. Sprinkle with cayenne pepper and mix to combine.

3. Finally add chopped kale to skillet. Cook for another 2-3 minutes, until kale has wilted and gone a brighter green colour.

4. Veg can be replaced with whatever you have on hand. I like this recipe to use up any sad looking vegetables I have handy. Broccoli and spinach are also delicious, as well as cauliflower and carrot.

5. If you don't have cooked quinoa this can be done while you're satueeing your veg. Add 1 cup quinoa to 2 cups water, bring to boil and let simmer for 15 minutes. Or until cooked. Save any leftover quinoa to top on salads, or buddha bowls, or try my Creamy Quinoa Porridge for breakfast.

11. The Ultimate Baked Falafels

Prep Time: 20 Minutes

Cook Time: 15 Minutes

Servings: 5

Ingredients

- 1/4 cup old-fashioned rolled oats
- 1/2 cup fresh parsley
- 6 cloves garlic
- 1 small onion
- 1 can chickpeas (strained and rinsed)
- 2 tbsp nutritional yeast
- 2 tbsp tahini
- 1/2 lemon juiced
- 1 tbsp olive oil
- 1/2 tsp ground cumin
- 1/2 tsp ground coriander
- 1/4 tsp ground cardamom
- 1/2 tsp sea salt
- 1/4 tsp pepper

- pinch cayenne pepper
- 2 tbsp olive oil (for painting)

For The Citrus Tahini Dressing:

- 1/4 cup tahini
- 2 lemons juices
- pinch salt
- filtered water , to thin (I used 2-3 tbsp)
- 5 whole-grain tortilla wraps
- 1 cup mixed greens of choice
- 1 cup purple cabbage , thinly sliced
- 1/2 cup cucumber , thinly sliced
- 2 avocados , thinly sliced

Instructions

1. In your food processor add oats, pulse into a flour-like substance. Remove from food processor and place to the side.
2. Next add parsley, garlic and onion to food processor. Pulse until finely chopped. Then add oat flour, chickpeas, nutritional yeast, tahini, lemon juice, olive oil, cumin, coriander, cardamom, sea salt, pepper and a pinch cayenne pepper. Pulse until it becomes a crumbly dough-like texture.
3. Transfer falafel dough to mixing bowl. Preheat oven to 375F/190C. Line a baking tray with parchment paper and scoop rounded tablespoon amounts of dough onto parchment paper, and gently form balls. (I used an ice cream scoop to do this.)
4. Paint falafels with a bit of olive oil and place in the oven to bake for 15-20 minutes, or until golden in colour.
5. To make the Citrus Tahini Sauce: in a bowl add tahini, lemon juice and salt. Mix to combine. Add splashes of water to thin until you've reached desired consistency. (I used 2-3 tbsp). Drizzle falafels with tahini sauce for eating.

6. To make the wraps combine mixed greens, cabbage, cucumber, avocado and 2-3 falafels in a whole wheat tortilla wrap, drizzle with citrus tahini dressing and serve.

Prep Time: 15 Minutes

Cook Time: 30 Minutes

Servings: 4

Ingredients

- 1 small cooking pumpkin (550g) or red kuri squash, kabocha squash, or butternut squash
- 2 tbsp neutral oil
- 1 tsp pumpkin pie spice (or quatre épices)
- 1/2 tsp cardamom
- 2 cloves garlic finely chopped
- pinch sea salt
- 5 oz baby greens (140 g) i.e. baby spinach, kale or lambs lettuce
- 1/2 cup green beans chopped
- 1/4 cup pomegranate seeds
- 1 avocado cut into cubes
- 1/4 cup hazelnuts
- 4 tbsp balsamic vinegar
- 2 tbsp extra virgin olive oil
- 1/8 tsp sea salt

- 1/8 tsp pepper

Instructions

1. Preheat oven to 400F/200C. Chop cooking pumpkin into bite sized pieces. (If using butternut squash, peel skin). In a small bowl add neutral oil, pumpkin pie spice, cardamom, garlic and sea salt. Whisk to combine. Drizzle mixture over pumpkin in a large mixing bowl, and toss to combine.
2. Line a baking tray with parchment paper and transfer pumpkin to tray. Spread pumpkin out so its not crowded (you might need two trays for this). Bake for 25 minutes, or until golden and cooked through. (Flip pumpkin pieces with spatula halfway through to ensure all sides are evenly roasted).
3. While you're waiting for the pumpkin to cook finely chop parsley and place to the side. Toast hazelnuts by chopping and adding to a skillet, bring to medium-high heat and toast, stirring often, until browned and aromatic.
4. In a large mixing bowl add roasted pumpkin, salad greens, chopped green beans, pomegranate seeds, and avocado. Drizzle with quality balsamic and olive oil.

Season with salt and pepper and toss gently to combine. Sprinkle salad with toasted hazelnuts and serve.

Prep Time: 15 Minutes

Cook Time: 20 Minutes

Servings: 2

Ingredients

Buddha Bowl:

- 1 heaping cup quinoa, cooked
- 1 handful baby greens (spinach or lambs lettuce)
- 1/4 cup cucumber, chopped
- 1/2 zucchini, spirazlied or grated
- 1/3 cup purple cabbage, thinly sliced
- 1/2 cup edamame beans
- 1 avocado

Mustard Paprika Dressing:

- 2 tbsp olive oil
- 2 tbsp apple cider vinegar
- 2 tsp dijon mustard
- 1 clove garlic , finely chopped
- 1/2 tsp paprika
- pinch salt

Instructions

1. Prepare the veg: chop cucumber, spiralize zucchini using a spiralizer (or grate with a cheese grater), thinly slice cabbage using a mandoline or a sharp knife. If using frozen edamame, steam for 3-5 minutes until al-dente.

2. Between two bowls, divide cooked quinoa, leafy greens, cucumber, zucchini, cabbage, edamame beans, and avocado.

3. Prepare dressing by mixing oil, apple cider vinegar, mustard, diced garlic, paprika and salt. Stir well with a fork to combine. Pour dressing over buddha bowl, using as much as desired.

4. To make 1 cup cooked quinoa: combine 1/3 cup quinoa and 2/3 cup water in a pot. Bring to a boil, then reduce heat and simmer for 12-15 minutes.

5. I like to prepare a big batch of quinoa to last me through the week, so it's ready for buddha bowls like this. Quinoa will keep in fridge for up to one week.

6. Mustard Paprika Dressing will keep in fridge for up to 5 days.

7. I've used a spiralizer to make my zucchini into noodles, however it's not necessary for this recipe. If

you don't have one simply grate the zucchini using a cheese grater.

8. I've used a mandoline to thinly slice my cabbage, however it's not necessary for this recipe. If you don't have one simply slice the cabbage very thinly with a sharp knife.

Prep Time: 20 Minutes

Cook Time: 50 Minutes

Servings: 8

Ingredients

- 1 butternut squash (about 2 lb)
- 2 sweet potato
- 3 tbsp avocado oil (or other neutral oil)
- 1/8 tsp sea salt
- 1/8 tsp pepper
- 1 white onion
- 3 cloves garlic
- 1 tbsp avocado oil (or other neutral oil)
- 4 cups vegetable broth , plus more if needed
- 1 tbsp curry powder
- 1/2 tsp cumin
- 1/4 tsp paprika
- 1/4 tsp ginger
- 1/4 tsp cayenne pepper (optional)
- 1 can coconut milk (400 ml/14 fl oz. can)
- 1/3 cup peanuts , for garnish (optional)

- kale chips , for garnish (optional)

Instructions

1. Preheat oven to 400F/200C. Peel and chop butternut squash into small bit sized cubes. Chop sweet potato into bite sized cubes. Add veg to a baking dish and drizzle with oil. Sprinkle generously with sea salt and pepper and cook for 30 minutes, or until cooked through.

2. Dice onion and garlic and add to a large pot with pinch sea salt. Drizzle with 1 tbsp oil and bring to medium-low heat. Simmer on low, until onion turns translucent in colour (10 mins). Add roasted squash and sweet potato and pour in vegetable broth.

3. Bring to simmer and add spices: curry powder, cumin, paprika, ginger and cayenne. Cook for another 10-20 minutes. Puree soup with hand mixer, or transfer to blender to puree in batches. (Optional to add splashes more broth if needed for blending if it's too thick, but I didn't need to). Pour canned coconut milk into pureed soup to finish, stir to combine.

4. In a skillet toast peanuts on medium-high heat until browned and fragrant (approx. 5 minutes). Make kale

chips for garnish (recipe link in notes. Takes 5 minutes).

5. Pour soup into bowls and top with roasted peanuts and kale chips. Season with sea salt and pepper.

Prep Time: 20 Minutes

Cook Time: 15 Minutes

Servings: 4

Ingredients

- 1 cup quinoa uncooked
- 2 cups water
- 1/2 tsp turmeric powder
- pinch sea salt
- 1 cup edamame beans
- 1 zucchini spiralized
- 1 cup carrot grated
- 1 cup cooked beetroot chopped
- 1 avocado chopped
- 1/4 cucumber thinly sliced
- 1/2 cup hummus

For The Garlic-Tahini Dressing:

- 1/4 cup tahini
- 2 limes juice
- 2 cloves garlic finely chopped

- pinch salt and pepper
- 2 tbsp water to thin

Instructions

1. Start by cooking quinoa. In a saucepan add 1 cup quinoa to 2 cups water. Bring to a boil then reduce heat, add turmeric and pinch sea salt, and simmer for 12-15 minutes or until cooked and pillowy.
2. Spiralize zucchini (or grate it), and grate carrots, chop beetroot, and thinly slice avocado and cucumber.
3. Divide quinoa, edamame, zucchini, carrots, beetroot, avocado and cucumber between bowls. Divide hummus between each bowl.
4. Prepare dressing: In a small bowl add 1/4 cup tahini, the juice of 2 limes, finely chopped garlic, and pinch salt and pepper. Whisk to combine. Add splashes of water as desired for thinning, I used about 2 tablespoons. Drizzle over buddha bowls and serve.

Prep Time: 20 Minutes

Cook Time: 15 Minutes

Servings: 4

Ingredients

- 2 cups chickpeas
- 3 tbsp tahini
- 1 lemon juiced
- 1/4 cup red onion finely chopped
- 1/4 tsp sea salt
- 1/4 tsp pepper
- 8 slices whole wheat bread
- 4 tsp dijon mustard
- 1/3 cup cucumber thinly sliced
- 1/2 cup purple cabbage thinly sliced
- 1/2 cup alfalfa sprouts

Instructions

1. In a food processor (or blender), pulse chickpeas a few times to break into small pieces, (you can also use the

back of a fork or potato masher). Transfer to mixing bowl.

2. In a small bowl combine tahini and the juice of one lemon. Mix to combine, then add to mashed chickpeas. Add diced onion, sea salt and pepper and stir to combine. Optional to add more salt, pepper and lemon juice for desired taste.

3. Build four sandwiches by adding 1 tsp dijon mustard to each (spread to even), chickpea tuna, cucumber, red cabbage, and alfalfa sprouts. Season with more salt and pepper, and close with slice of bread.

Prep Time: 20 Minutes

Cook Time: 15 Minutes

Servings: 4

Ingredients

Sauce:

- 1/4 cup tamari or soy sauce
- 2 tbsp sesame oil
- 1 tbsp rice vinegar
- 2 tsp maple syrup
- 1 tsp ginger grated
- 1/4 tsp siracha plus more if desired

Other:

- 1 packet soy bean noodles 8 oz/200g (or buckwheat noodles, rice noodles, ramen)
- 2 cloves garlic
- 2 cups cremini mushrooms chopped
- 1 tbsp coconut oil
- 1 red bell pepper
- 2 carrots

- 1/2 cup red cabbage shredded

- 2 green onions chopped

- 1/3 cup cilantro chopped, tightly packed (optional)

Instructions

1. Start by preparing your sauce and cooking your noodles. In a small bowl combine tamari, sesame oil, rice vinegar, maple syrup, grated ginger and siracha. Whisk together and place to the side.

2. Bring a pot of water to boil and add soybean noodles, cook for 2-4 minutes, or as directed on package until just aldente. Strain and rinse with cold water.

3. In a deep skillet add garlic, mushrooms and coconut oil. Cook on medium heat for 10 minutes, until softened. Thinly slice bell pepper and cut carrots jullien style with a mandoline (alternitively, grate carrots with a box grater). Add bell pepper, carrots and cabbage to skillet and cook until slightly wilted (5-10 minutes).

4. Add noodles to the skillet and pour in sauce. Toss everything to combine. Serve in bowls sprinkled with green onion and cilantro to top.

Prep Time: 10 Minutes

Cook Time: 15 Minutes

Servings: 4

Ingredients

- 3 shallots (or 1 yellow onion), chopped
- 4 cloves garlic diced
- 1 tbsp coconut oil
- 1.5 cups raw cashews preferably soaked for 1 hr, strained
- 2 cups almond milk
- 1/4 cup nutritional yeast
- 2 tbsp lemon juice (about 1/2 lemon)
- 1 1/2 tsp sea salt
- 1/2 tsp pepper
- 1/2 tsp paprika
- 3/4 cup parsley curly, finely chopped (optional)
- 1/2 tsp cayenne pepper flakes to sprinkle (optional)

For The Pasta

- 1 package gluten-free spaghetti noodles (500g/17.6 oz)

Instructions

1. Bring a skillet to medium heat, add chopped shallots (or onion), garlic and coconut oil. Cook until softened (5-10 mins).
2. Transfer garlic and onion to a blender with raw cashews (strained), almond milk, nutritional yeast, lemon juice, sea salt, pepper and paprika. Blend until smooth.
3. To make pasta: bring a pot of water to a boil and add noodles. Cook as directed on package, until al-dente (typically 7-9 minutes). Strain and transfer noodles back to pot. Pour Alfredo sauce over noodles and mix to combine. Taste, season with more sea salt and pepper as desired. Optional to add chopped parsley, stir to combine, and cayenne pepper flakes to taste.
4. Soaking raw cashews in advance is preferred for smoother and creamier consistency. Although it's not necessary. The recipe will still work without soaking. I like to soak my cashews for at least two hour, or

overnight. Speed up soak time to 1 hour by pouring boiling water into bowl of cashews.

5. Do ahead: Vegan Alfredo sauce can be made in advance, and will keep in fridge for up to 5 days. When ready to use, warm in sauce pan or microwave.

6. Freeze this recipe: Vegan Alfredo sauce can be frozen in an air tight container for up to one month. Let thaw before using. When ready to use, warm in saucepan or microwave.

7. Make it nut free: by subbing hemp hearts for cashews (no soaking necessary). Sub soy or oat milk for almond milk.

Prep Time: 20 Minutes

Cook Time: 10 Minutes

Servings: 6

Ingredients

- 5 cup chickpea pasta
- pinch sea salt
- 1-2 tbsp sesame oil
- 1 cup purple cabbage shredded
- 1 cup carrots grated
- 1 cup cucumber chopped
- 4 green onions chopped
- 1/3 cup peanuts chopped
- 1/3 cup cilantro chopped

For The Peanut Sauce:

- 1/4 cup + 2 tbsp all-natural peanut butter
- 1/4 cup water
- 3 tbsp rice vinegar
- 2 tbsp tamari
- 2 tbsp maple syrup

- 1 tbsp sesame oil
- 1 clove garlic
- 1/4 tsp cayenne pepper

Instructions

1. In a large pot bring water to boil. Add a generous pinch of sea salt and pour in pasta. Cook chickpea pasta until just al-dente (about 3 minutes. Pasta will continue to cook as it cools).
2. Strain pasta and rinse with cold water. Place back in pot, drizzle with sesame oil and stir gently. Cover with a tea towel and let cool.
3. In a large mixing bowl add shredded cabbage, carrots, chopped cucumber,
4. and onions. Add cooked pasta.
5. Prepare peanut sauce in a small bowl by whisking together peanut butter, water, rice vinegar, tamari, maple syrup, sesame oil, garlic and cayenne.
6. Pour peanut sauce over pasta salad and mix gently to combine. Sprinkle
7. with green onion, peanuts, and cilantro. Mix again.

Prep Time: 20 Minutes

Cook Time: 10 Minutes

Servings: 6

Ingredients

- 2/3 cup quinoa
- 1 1/2 cup water
- 1/2 cup almonds chopped
- 1 shallot small
- 1 cup carrots grated
- 1 can chickpeas (14 fl oz/400 ml)
- 2.5 oz arugula (70 g)
- 1/2 cup mint tightly packed
- 1/4 cup dates chopped

Moroccan Salad Dressing:

- 1/4 cup + 2 tbsp olive oil
- 2 tbsp lemon juice
- 2 tbsp orange juice
- 1 tbsp maple syrup
- 1/2 tsp cinnamon

- 1/2 tsp ginger
- 1/2 tsp cumin
- 1/2 tsp coriander
- 1/4 tsp sea salt
- pinch red pepper flakes

Instructions

1. In a saucepan combine quinoa and water. Bring to a boil, then reduce to simmer and cook quinoa for 12-15 minutes. Fluff with a spoon and cover with tea towel. Let cool.
2. Toast almonds in a skillet on medium heat, stirring often until fragrant and golden browned (approx. 8-10 mins). Remove from heat.
3. Prepare dressing in a small bowl by whisking together oil, lemon juice, orange juice, maple syrup, cinnamon, ginger, cumin, coriander, sea salt and red pepper flakes.
4. In a large mixing bowl combine quinoa, chopped shallot, grated carrot, chickpeas, arugula, chopped mint and dates and toasted almonds. Pour over dressing and toss to combine

21. Black Bean Stuffed Sweet Potatoes

Prep Time: 15 Minutes

Cook Time: 40 Minutes

Servings: 6

Ingredients

- 4 sweet potatoes
- 1 tbsp olive oil or avocado oil
- 1 1/2 cups black beans
- 1 cup cherry tomatoes chopped
- 1/2 cup corn
- 1/3 cup cilantro chopped, tightly packed
- 1/4 cup red onion diced
- 1 clove garlic diced
- 1/2 lime juiced
- 2 tsp olive oil
- 1/4 tsp sea salt
- pinch pepper
- pinch chili flakes

Easy Guacamole (For Topping)

- 1 avocado

- 2 tsp lime juice

- pinch sea salt

Vegan Sour Cream (To Drizzle)

- 1/3 cup coconut yogurt

- 1/2 tsp lime juice

- pinch sea salt

Instructions

1. Preheat oven to 400F/200C. Using a fork, poke small holes in sweet potatoes going all the way round, about 1-inch apart. Line baking tray with parchment paper, and paint sweet potatoes with oil to lightly coat. Bake for 40 minutes to 1 hour, or until fork tender. (See notes to check for doneness).

2. In a bowl combine the black beans, tomato, corn, cilantro, red onion and garlic. Drizzle with the lime juice and olive oil. Sprinkle with sea salt, pepper and chili flakes. Mix to combine.

3. Prepare easy guacamole: Mash avocado in a bowl with lime juice and a pinch of sea salt.

4. Prepare vegan sour cream: In a separate bowl mix together coconut yogurt, lime juice and sea salt.

5. Cut sweet potatoes in half and fill with black bean medley. Top with easy guacamole and drizzle with vegan sour cream.

Prep Time: 20 Minutes

Cook Time: 40 Minutes

Servings: 6

Ingredients

- 2 cups red cabbage shredded
- 2 cups white cabbage shredded
- 1 cup carrots grated (about 2 carrots)
- 1 cup broccolini (or traditional broccoli florets) chopped
- 1 cup cilantro finely chopped
- 1/2 cup parsley finely chopped
- 1/4 cup peanuts chopped
- 4 green onions

Peanut Dressing:

- 1/4 cup olive oil
- 1/4 cup apple cider vinegar
- 1/4 cup peanut butter
- 1 clove garlic finely chopped
- 1 tbsp tamari or soy sauce, or coconut aminos

- 1 tbsp agave

- 1 tbsp ginger fresh, grated

- 1/2 tsp sea salt

- 1/4 tsp chili flakes

Instructions

1. Using a food processor, thinly slice red and white cabbage, and grate carrots. (Alternately, thinly slice cabbage with a sharp knife and grate carrot with a box grater). Finely chop the broccoli florets, cilantro, parsley and peanuts. Thinly slice green onion. Add everything to a large mixing bowl.

2. In a separate smaller bowl combine dressing ingredients: olive oil, apple cider vinegar, peanut butter, garlic, tamari, agave, ginger, sea salt and chili flakes. Whisk to combine.

3. Pour dressing over slaw and toss to combine. Chill in fridge until ready to serve.

Prep Time: 30 Minutes

Cook Time: 20 Minutes

Servings: 12

Ingredients

- 3 cups water
- 2 cups uncooked sushi rice
- 1/2 cup rice vinegar
- 1/4 cup white sugar
- 1 tsp salt
- 1 tbsp sesame oil
- coconut oil for moulding
- 1 mango
- 1 avocado
- tamari to dip (for savoury sushi donuts)
- 1/2 can coconut milk to dip (for sweet sushi donuts)
- 1 tbsp agave to dip (for sweet sushi donuts)

Instructions

1. And water and rice to a pot and bring to boil. Then reduce heat to simmer, cover with a lid, and cook for 20 minutes, or until cooked through.

2. Meanwhile, in a saucepan combine rice vinegar, sugar, salt and sesame oil. Bring to low heat and stir to combine.

3. When rice is cooked remove pour in the liquid mixture in batches, stirring rice to combine.

4. Cover rice with clean dish towel and let sit for 10-15 minutes. Then scoop rice onto a clean surface or wide bowl and spread out to cool slightly before handling.

5. Thinly slice avocado and mango. When rice is cool enough to handle lather donut moulds with a bit of coconut oil. (I used a 6-cavity silicon donut mould for this). Scoop rice into donut moulds to fill. Then inverse mould onto a flat surface to remove donut shapes. (If your hands are sticking to the rice, wet hands with water and continue).

6. Decorate each donut with avocado or mango. Serve with tamari to dip for the avocado sushi donuts. In a small bowl, whisk together coconut milk and agave. Serve as dip for the mango donuts.

Prep Time: 30 Minutes

Cook Time: 20 Minutes

Servings: 6

Ingredients

- 1 cup homemade vegan queso (or use store-bought)
- 1 tbsp coconut oil
- 12 oz plant-based ground
- 4 tsp taco seasoning
- 6 large 10-inch tortillas
- 6 small 5-inch tortillas (or two more 10-inch tortillas cut into quarters).
- 1-2 cups tortilla chips
- ½ cup salsa
- ½ cup chopped tomatoes
- 1 cup iceberg lettuce grated
- ¼ cup cilantro leaves chopped
- 2 avocados mashed
- olive oil for drizzling

Instructions

1. If using the homemade Vegan Queso, make this now. (Alternatively you can use store-bought).

2. Melt the coconut oil in a large skillet on medium-heat, then add the plant-based ground and taco seasoning. Cook until browned and combined, about 5 to 7 mins. Transfer to a bowl and side aside. Prepare all your ingredients, if you haven't already for building.

3. Build the crunchwrap: Place a large tortilla on a work surface. Layer the centre with a bit of vegan queso leaving about 1.5-2 inches around the edges for folding. Then top the next layer with plant-based ground, nachos (placed side-by-side with the tip facing inwards to make a circle shape), salsa, chopped tomatoes, lettuce, cilantro and smashed avocado.

4. *(See images in the blog post under, "How to Make a Crunchwrap Supreme," for a visual, if helpful).

5. Top with the small tortilla and fold in the edges of the large tortilla over to close.

6. (If using only 10-inch tortillas, instead of the small 5-inch tortillas, cut a 10-inch tortilla into quarters and place a quarter piece into the centre of your crunchwrap. Fold in the edges of the large tortilla over to close).

7. Heat a drizzle of olive oil in the large (cleaned) skillet on medium heat and place the crunchwrap seam-side down, cook for 2 to 3 minutes until the exterior is firm and golden brown, flip and cook the other side until golden. Cut and serve.

8. Continue making crunchwraps in Step 3, 4 and 5 until you've used all the ingredients.

Prep Time: 15 Minutes

Cook Time: 10 Minutes

Servings: 6

Ingredients

- 2 cups cauliflower florets
- 2 tbsp coconut oil
- 1 shallot finely chopped
- 2 cloves garlic finely chopped
- 1 1/2 cup unsweetened almond milk
- 1/4 cup nutritional yeast
- 1 tbsp dijon mustard
- 1 tbsp white miso
- 1 tsp fine sea salt
- pinch turmeric (optional for colour)
- 1 cup cashews
- pinch pepper for sprinkling
- pinch paprika for sprinkling (optional)
- 1 lb macaroni noodles

Instructions

1. Chop the cauliflower florets into small pieces and set aside. Bring a large pot of water to a boil (for the macaroni noodles).

2. Melt the coconut oil in a large deep skillet on medium heat. Add the chopped shallot and garlic and cook to soften, 5 mins. Pour in the almond milk, nutritional yeast, dijon mustard, miso, sea salt and turmeric. Bring to a simmer on medium-high heat and whisk to combine.

3. Add the chopped cauliflower florets and cashews into the skillet and simmer, with the lid on, until the cauliflower is very soft, 15 minutes. Transfer to a high speed blender and blend until smooth. Then pour the cheese sauce back into the skillet.

4. Meanwhile, cook the pasta noodles until al-dente, about 7 mins. Scoop the cooked noodles into the skillet with the sauce and mix everything to combine. Serve in bowls and sprinkle with pepper and paprika.

Prep Time: 15 Minutes

Cook Time: 25 Minutes

Servings: 6

Ingredients

- 1 yellow onion finely chopped
- 2 cloves garlic
- 1 tbsp coconut oil
- 1 lb cremini mushrooms (16 oz), sliced
- 340 g Plant-Based Ground (optional)
- 1.5 cups vegetable broth
- ½ can coconut milk (200 ml)
- 2 tbsp nutritional yeast
- 1 tbsp tamari
- 1 tbsp lemon juice
- 1 tbsp Dijon mustard
- ¼ tsp sea salt finely ground
- pinch pepper
- ¼ cup all-purpose flour
- 500 g pasta noodles of choice I used Pappardelle

Instructions

1. In a large deep skillet add the onion, garlic and coconut oil. Bring to medium heat and cook until softened. Add the mushrooms and continue cooking until the mushrooms are softened and browned (about 10 mins). If using the plant-based ground, add it to the skillet and cook until browned (about 7 mins). Remove from heat.

2. In a small saucepan, whisk together the vegetable broth, coconut milk, nutritional yeast, tamari, lemon juice, Dijon mustard, sea salt and pepper on low heat. Pour the liquid mixture into the skillet reserving ½ cup of the liquid. Add the all-purpose flour to the reserved liquid and whisk to combine. Then add the reserved liquid to the skillet and stir everything to combine. Increase heat to a low simmer.

3. Add the pasta noodles to a large pot of boiling water. Cook until al-dente (about 7 mins). Strain and gently rinse with cold water, then add the pasta to the skillet and toss together to combine.

Prep Time: 30 Minutes

Cook Time: 25 Minutes

Servings: 6

Ingredients

Cashew Cheese:

- 1 ½ cups raw cashews soaked and strained
- 1 cup water
- 2 cloves garlic
- ¼ cup nutritional yeast
- 3 tbsp lemon juice
- 2 tbsp arrowroot starch or tapioca starch, or corn starch
- 1 tsp onion powder
- ½ tsp sea salt

Pasta and Everything Else:

- 2 tbsp olive oil
- 1 yellow onion finely chopped
- 2 red bell peppers finely chopped
- ¼ tsp sea salt

- 12 oz Plant-Based ground (340 g) (or lentils)
- 23 fl oz tomato sauce (660 mL)
- 1 lb ziti noodles (450 g)
- 1 3/4 cup vegan mozzarella cheese (8 oz/200 g), shredded

Instructions

1. Prepare the cashew cheese: in a high-speed blender add the cashews, water, garlic, nutritional yeast, lemon juice, tapioca starch, onion powder and salt. Blend until smooth and creamy.

2. Drizzle the olive oil in a large deep skillet and bring to medium heat. Add the onion, bell peppers and sea salt. Cook until softened, about 10 mins. Add the vegan ground "beef" and cook, stirring often until browned, about 5 mins. Pour in the tomato sauce and bring to a low simmer.

3. Pre-heat oven to 375F/190C. Bring a large pot of water to a boil and add the ziti noodles. Cook until almost al-dente, about 6 mins (they should be just undercooked as they will continue cooking in the oven). Strain and add back to the pot. Scoop 1 cup of the tomato sauce and mix to combine.

4. Assemble the Ziti! Scoop 1 ½ cups of the tomato sauce into a large casserole dish (8x11 inches). Smooth with a spatula into an even layer. Next add the noodles, followed by the remaining tomato sauce, and finally drizzle with the cashew cheese to cover. To finish, sprinkle with the shredded cheese.

5. Place a baking tray on the bottom rack to catch any overspill, if any, and bake for 25 minutes until the cheese is melted and golden around the edges.

Prep Time: 30 Minutes

Cook Time: 30 Minutes

Servings: 4

Ingredients

- 1 cauliflower (small), chopped into bite-sized florets
- 2 zucchini chopped
- 3 tbsp avocado oil
- 1 yellow onion finely chopped
- 2 carrots chopped
- 1 tbsp turmeric
- 1 tsp curry powder
- 1 tsp cumin
- 1 tsp cinnamon
- 1 tsp ginger fresh, peeled and grated
- 1 can coconut milk
- 1/2 tsp sea salt finely ground, plus more if desired
- 1 can chickpeas strained and rinsed

Instructions

1. Preheat oven to 400F/200C. Add the chopped cauliflower and zucchini to a baking tray and drizzle with 2 tablespoons of avocado oil. Mix to combine. Cook for 25 to 30 minutes, or until cauliflower is fork tender.

2. Meanwhile, add the onion and carrots in a large deep skillet with 1 tablespoons of avocado oil. Cook on medium heat to soften (about 10 mins). Mix in the turmeric, curry powder, cumin, cinnamon, ginger and sea salt. Pour in the coconut milk. Mix to combine.

3. Add the cooked cauliflower and zucchini and pour in the chickpeas. Stir everything to combine. Optional to add more salt to taste. Keep on a low simmer until ready to eat. Serve with rice, quinoa or naan bread.

Prep Time: 15 Minutes

Cook Time: 30 Minutes

Servings: 4

Ingredients

- 1 cup cherry tomatoes
- 1 tbsp avocado oil or other neutral oil
- 1 packet pasta of choice (500g)
- 1/3 cup olive oil
- 1/4 cup lemon juice
- 1 cup corn
- 1 cup chickpeas
- 1/4 cup chives chopped
- 1/4 cup fresh parsley chopped
- 1/4 cup mint leaves chopped
- 1/4 cup basil chopped
- 1/4 tsp sea salt
- 1/4 tsp cayenne pepper optional

Instructions

1. Preheat oven to 200C /400F. Paint cherry tomatoes with avocado oil and bake for 15 mins, or until bright and bursted. Remove from oven and place to the side.

2. Bring a large pot of water to a boil. Add noodles and cook spaghetti until just al-dente (approx. 5 minutes). Strain noodles.

3. Transfer noodles back to pot and drizzle with olive oil and lemon juice. Add tomatoes and corn, chickpeas, and chopped chives, parsley, mint and basil. Sprinkle with sea salt and cayenne (optional). Toss to combine.

Prep Time: 30 Minutes

Cook Time: 50 Minutes

Servings: 6

Ingredients

- 6 bell peppers
- 1 tbsp coconut oil
- 3 cloves garlic finely chopped
- 1 yellow onion finely chopped
- 1 tomato chopped
- Pinch sea salt plus more for sprinkling
- Pinch pepper plus more for sprinkling
- 12 oz Vegan ground beef , such as Beyond Beef, Yves or Lightlife Plant-based Ground (or 1.5 cups green/brown lentils)
- 1 teaspoon Italian seasoning
- 1 cup cooked rice
- 1 cup tomato sauce
- 1/3 cup Homemade Vegan Mozzarella , or store-bought
- Fresh basil chopped, to sprinkle

Instructions

1. Preheat oven to 400F/200C. Cut the tops off the bell peppers and scoop out the core and inner seeds. Nuzzle the bell peppers into a rectangular baking dish (9 x 13-inch).

2. In a saucepan combine the coconut oil, garlic, onion, tomato, a generous pinch of sea salt and pepper. Cook until softened and the onion turns translucent, about 10 minutes. Add the vegan ground beef (or lentils) and Italian seasoning and cook until browned. Pour in the rice and the tomato sauce. Stir to combine.

3. Stuff the bell peppers with filling and top each with mozzarella cheese. Sprinkle with more sea salt and pepper. Cover the baking dish with foil (or reusable cover) and cook for 40 minutes, or until the peppers are tender. Remove foil and cook for another 10 minutes, until the cheese is bubbly. Sprinkle with fresh basil and serve.

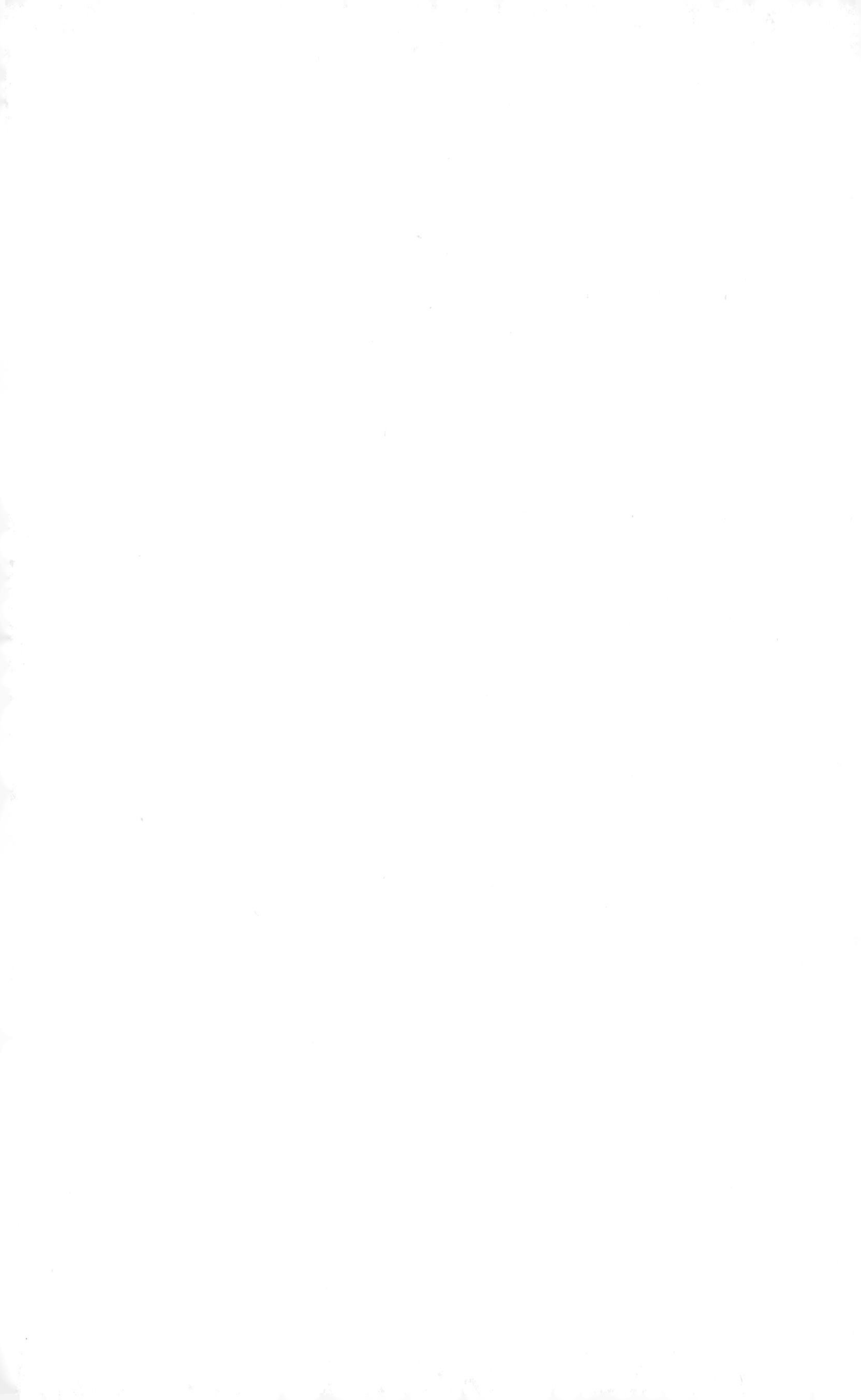